LOSE
WEIGHT
AND KEEP IT OFF
FOR GOOD

Marva Riley

LOST WEIGHT and keep it off for good!
© 2022 Marva Riley.

ISBN: 979-8-218-12557-8 (sc)
ISBN: 979-8-218-12558-5 (hc)
Imprint: MarvaRiley

Editing: Karen Yvonne Hamilton, Yesterday Press
www.yesterdaypress.com Jupiter, Florida

Cover Design & Layout:
Susan Gulash, Creative Director/Owner, *Gulash Graphics*
www.gulashgraphics.com

LOSE WEIGHT
and keep it off for good

(No more yo-yo dieting. Tried and proven sustainable weight loss
strategies to help you to succeed at becoming and remaining the
Healthiest Version of Yourself)

HEALTHY WEIGHT LOSS
NO MORE YO-YO DIETING
12 Steps to Achieving your ideal weight and keeping it off for
good.

Also written by Marva Riley, RN

Eat Sleep Meditate A Nurse's Guide to Health
SHEIR: Simple Healthy Easy Inexpensive Recipes

This book is not intended to be a substitute for medical care or advice from your healthcare provider / doctor. You should consult with your physician before making any changes to your diet and exercise.

To my beautiful grandson Asa
Asa, which means Doctor, Healer
The one who will join me in speaking healings to the worlds.

— Table of Contents —

3 Tiers to Sustained Weight Loss

— Table of Contents —

Recipes

—Prologue—

January 2nd is the day when everyone is deciding to set their New year's Fitness goals and resolutions. If you are a regular gym member, frustration and anger are perhaps words that you might use to discuss how you feel during the months of January to March. This is when the New Year's resolution enthusiasts cram the gym, stuck to the treadmill, elliptical, or biceps machines, trying their best to live up to the unrealistic expectations that are often thrusted upon them by the weight loss industry. Trying their best to win the weight loss battle once and for all. To take back that smoking body they were once so proud of.

One by one, the enthusiasts fall off the bandwagon. Frustrated and feeling like a failure, they return to the so-called "bad habits" they really enjoyed.

By March, perhaps 50% of these well-intentioned devotees quit out of frustration and sometimes shame. The reasons they cite are that they feel like a failure and see no reason to continue trying. ABC Columbia states, "Research shows 80% of people abandon their New Year's resolutions by February" (Dec 31, 2021 5:23 PM EST by CNN)

Many have gone down this road more than once. Many have put 100% in on day one. Research has shown that 80% fail by day ninety. Why is that?

This cycle goes on every year. The gym fanatics and die-hard health and fitness enthusiasts know that. So, with bated breath, they wait till March 31st to take back their rightful place in the gym, at the park, or wherever fitness zealots hang out.

Why the craze about weight loss and why new year's resolutions?

Fitness, health, weight loss, weight loss products, gyms, and even some parks are huge businesses. According to Businesswire.com, "the U.S. weight loss market reached a record of $78 billion in 2019." "The weight loss market is forecast to grow 2.6% annually through 2023", according to John LaRosa at Marketresearch.com.

So, you see, weight loss is a big business. Advertisements start late fall to early winter, and peak around Christmas to New Year. This is the time when folks are in the mood to spend without much thought of the expenses.

We are prompted, tempted, cajoled, and made to feel guilty in an effort to convince us to buy gym memberships, home gym equipment, weight loss products including pills, shakes, waist trimmers, etc through ads on TV, social media, magazines, the Internet, newspapers and weight loss business people.

Personal trainers are busy putting together packages to convince us to hire their well-needed services.
These ads are persuasive because who doesn't want to look like the buffed guy or the skinny chick we see in these commercials every few seconds?

Like I did in the past, many succumb to the temptation and pressure, as we hand over our credit cards for that gym membership, for that equipment, home gym, and products. Emotional buying! Most never cancel that gym membership, although they have not been there in years. They feel shame and perhaps think that canceling the gym membership is an indication of failure. Month after month that $20, $50 or $150 is deducted from their credit card without any thought of canceling. Besides, the gyms make it difficult and inconvenient to cancel. They can sign up for the gym online, BUT, you must go in to cancel. It's inconvenient and somehow, paying that monthly gym fee makes them feel better. Makes them feel like they are doing something about their health.

Soon these well-intentioned treadmills, stationary bikes, ellipticals, and home gyms become closets as the gyms continue to deduct that monthly payment from their credit cards, although they have not entered that place in months, even years. What a waste of money. Out of frustration, the feeling of "I can't" takes hold of their minds. They give up, believing that voice in their heads as they return to their familiar habits and lifestyles.   The cycle continues.

According to ABC Columbia in 2021, "Research shows that 80% of people abandon their new year's resolution by February."

If you are in that 80%, there is no shame. You are not alone, **BUT,** I can reassure you that this is not the end of your story. YOU can be a part of that 20% who set the goal to get healthy and stay healthy. To get fit and stay fit. To lose that extra weight and keep it off for good. **To become the healthiest version of your beautiful self.** To love and be proud of the way you look and feel. To fit in that dress, pants, shirt, or bathing suit you've been longing to fit in.

I want to reassure you that it is NOT as complex as you think. The steps to sustained weight loss are very simple and doable. I would like to show you how.

Yes, you've probably heard this before, but I do know the secret to losing that weight and keeping it off for good!

I too was overweight with multiple health issues. I learned a few simple steps, tried them consistently, and they have helped me to enjoy the best shape that I have ever been in. As a young and as a middle-aged adult, I struggled with weight loss and tried many weight loss programs including shakes and pills. I would lose a ton of weight, however, as soon as I started eating real food again, I would regain the weight and then some.

Yes, I do know the secret to sustained weight loss, and I would like to show you how.

It's quite simple!

Keep reading!

Testimonials

Althea L. Essue
Certified Personal Trainer, Licensed Massage Therapist

I was born in the Caribbean, Jamaica to be exact. My family didn't have the privilege to own a car, so wherever I went, I had to walk. We didn't have a lot of money, so the foods I ate were planted/ grown by my family. We didn't have a refrigerator, so everything we ate was fresh and homemade. We didn't have electricity, so there was no television in the house. We were not allowed to stay in the house because we would make it dirty, so we had to go outside and play. I thought I was invincible. I thought I would always be forever young. I ate what I wanted, whenever I wanted and how much I wanted. Due to my age, I was able to be more active which kept my metabolism working optimally. I did that all throughout my adolescence, teenage years and well into my twenties.

I began my family during my mid-twenties and realized very quickly that I did not have as much time for myself as I did before getting married and having children. There were the late-night feedings, changing the diapers, cooking, house cleaning and a full-time job. I slowly adapted a lifestyle of doing more for others and less for myself. This went on for years and I didn't even realize what was happening.

My days consisted of waking up at 5:30am, preparing the children for day-care and school, dropping them off and then going to work. Notice, no where did I state that preparing my meals, having a healthy breakfast, taking a break to relax or to eat lunch away from my desk, going to the gym or taking a walk after work. My days were so busy, and I was trying to be Superwoman, trying to have the "Perfect Life" and the "American Dream", that I didn't realize that I was heading for disaster.

I was never taught to take care of myself first, and then my family.

12

As a woman from the Caribbean, I was taught to go to school, get a good education, get a good paying job, get married, have children, and always make sure that I had a great savings account and that my house was clean. I was told what to do, but not taught how to do it.

As I got older however, I started growing in ways that I was not liking or happy with. I continued to eat unhealthily. Because of my continuous busy life, I was eating late at night, eating processed foods, lots of white rice, white breads, and fried foods. It was what was available for the time or lack thereof. I became quite sedentary and was not visiting my doctor for my regular check-ups. I knew I was heading for disaster, but it was as if I couldn't stop.

Fast forward to 4 years ago when I had the wake-up call of my life. I was still overweight, still eating junk and barely active. In other words, I became content with being content. I would occasionally go to the gym, but I found excuses when I wasn't able to keep it consistent. Reasons I used for not eating healthy, staying stress free or being active:

1. I'm tired.

2. I can't miss my favorite show.

3. I can always order take-out from my favorite restaurant.

4. I can do it tomorrow (How many of us know that "To morrow never comes").

5. I just don't want to.

6. I can't miss the after work social (which consisted of eating fried foods and consuming alcohol and let's not forget about dessert.

 I could go on forever with the excuses because I chose not to take my health and my life more seriously.

Speaking of the wake-up call: You know when you go to the doctor, you give them authorization to call or email you with the results of your visit? I was waiting for the email to let me know that all my vitals were "normal". Instead, I received a phone call that I must make an appointment to come in to speak with the Doctor. This phone call literally "scared me straight".

As I drove to the Doctor's office, I began to imagine what was going to be discussed and I knew that it was not going to be a comfortable discussion. While sitting in the waiting room, I could feel my neck tensing up, getting the worst tension headache (more painful than a migraine) and I began to cry because I was scared. When I finally went into the examining room to speak with the Doctor, the news was horrible. I was told that I was borderline hypertensive, overweight and pre-diabetic. There was a simple fix to correct these health issues----change my diet (eating habits and food choices) and get off my couch, chair (at home and work) and move to save my life.

Easier said than done. I was sure that I could do this by myself because I was not used to asking for help. While attending church the following Sunday, I noticed one of my female friends looking very happy and a lot thinner than she was a few months ago. I worked up the courage to approach her and asked her what she was doing to transform into the happy, thinner, and powerful person that I was seeing. I wasn't prepared for the answer that she provided. She simply said, "I got someone to help me with eating healthier and exercising on a regular basis". I figured if she could do it, what was stopping me?

I dug deep down and adjusted my budget to include a personal trainer and eating real foods (fresh fruits and vegetables, water, etc.) I remember my first visit to the trainer. It was the second scariest time in my adult life. I had to have pictures taken of the real me; wearing only a sports bra and tights. I felt naked. When I looked at the pictures, I was shocked. That's when I decided that it was finally time to make a change. I took a step to change my future, and I never looked back.

I am now a Certified Personal Trainer. I work out 3-6 days a week; 3 days for myself personally and 3 days working out with two females that I train weekly. This is my way of giving back what was given to me. Paying it forward. I am dedicated to helping those who must get healthy in order to save their lives.

I am now comfortable and empowered to share my transformation and encourage you that you too can do it.

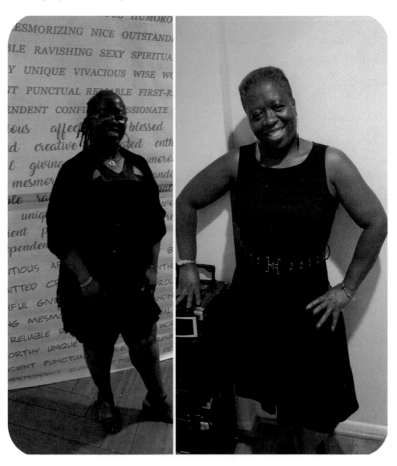

BEFORE & AFTER PICTURE
Althea L. Essue

LOSE WEIGHT AND KEEP IT OFF FOR GOOD

Yvonne P. Virtue, CAM
Director of Property Management, Avalon Property Management
Services

Ah! After years of yo-yo dieting; health coaches; trainers; multiple surgeries due to endometriosis; migraine headaches; and a litany of medications; I've finally had my Ah-hah moment and figured out how to develop a healthy lifestyle combining nutrition and exercise. It is not one or the other. It is both.

I've tried the quick fixes, pills and potions and failed miserably. Instead, applying a healthy dose of self-discipline, consistency, commitment, and focusing on the "WHY" has given me hope that weight management is achievable.

The WHY is engaging the brain in the process. Changing negative mindset and reprogramming bad habits resulting in amazing health.

For me it is daily self-talk. Developing a healthy relationship with food and exercise. Understanding that it is not a hobby but a lifestyle. So the process is slow and measurable. It is developing daily disciplines that will aid in reducing opportunities for diseases to ravish my body.

The best decision I ever made was seeing a health coach to deal with my emotional baggage. I spent three months just talking and detoxifying my mind. After those three months I was ready to begin my new health journey. I had a shift in my mindset.

My layman's approach is:

1. Design a meal plan for each day. Planning ahead keeps me focused, accountable and on track

2. Get a lunch bag. Everything I need to eat that day will be in that bag. This prevents me from purchasing fast food.

3. Learn to prepare healthy meals. I eat loads of fresh fruits and vegetables daily. I have a raw salad for lunch every day. There are plenty of resources available to help you in creating amazing healthy meals.

4. I have scheduled exercises at least three days per week including walking, lifting weights, cardio, jump ropes, However, on breaks at work, I do brisk walks, squats, stretches and anything to keep me active. I have a jump rope in my purse which comes in handy when time is an issue.

5. Drink lots of water. This is one area I struggle in so I try to drink at least 32 oz before I leave home in the mornings so it's easier to get another 32oz throughout the day.

6. Prayer and Meditation. I enjoy capturing photographs of nature, skies and water. I become totally gratitude-filled in the wonders of creation. This allows me to be still and refresh my mind.

7. Get a journal. I have been journaling since high school. I list things I'm grateful for and catalog my health journey. Some people weigh every day. I weigh once per week to just keep me on track. Do what works for you.

8. Have fun! I like to do puzzles, play my guitar, write songs, hang out at the beach, and watch the sun rise. Do something that makes you happy.

Now, my concern is not about how many pounds I've lost; that is the bonus. It's about staying focused every day on my nutrition and exercise. The result is that at 62 years old, I do not take any medication.

Marva Riley inspired me to try plant based nutrition, and that's the healthiest decision I've made in my entire life. I love her recipes in her recent book SHEIR. I'm healthier and loving it. I'm about 80% plant based. I do have fish and some chicken but am constantly working at reducing those.

Recently, my husband faced some health challenges with his prostate. We were encouraged to radically change our nutrition and focus on plant-based meals. After two months of plant-based nutrition, a biopsy revealed that there was no cancer.

I'm at a great place knowing that I can enjoy the process of a healthy lifestyle. No more stress and guilt. I am confident that if I mess up, I can reset and keep on moving.

This journey is not a sprint. It's slow and steady. No matter how much money one has, it cannot purchase health. So, let's commit to a lifetime of making healthy decisions. The rewards are eternal.

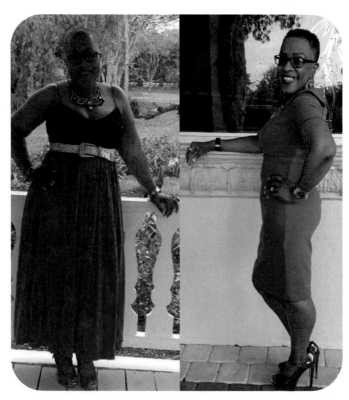

BEFORE & AFTER PICTURE
Yvonne P. Virtue, CAM

3 Tiers to Sustained Weight loss

MIND
SPIRIT
BODY

MIND. The Mind is where all change begins. As the Christian Bible states, "Be ye transformed by the renewing of your mind". You can shape your life by shaping your mind, your thoughts. Think about it, if you think you can, then you will. You will find a way. If you think you can't, you won't. You will make excuses.

A "Can Do" mindset is critical for success. This "can do" mindset gets your brain to focus on finding a way to make your goal happen.

SPIRIT. Fix your spirituality, fix your weight. A healthy life is a balanced life. We are not just our mind. We are not just our spirit. We are not just our body. We are all three in one. They all work together for our greater good.

BODY. The Christian Bible states, "You should know that **your body is a temple** for the Holy Spirit that you received from God and that lives in you. You don't own yourselves.," (1 Corinthians 6:19). You should know that approaching your weight loss goals are achievable if you approach it from a Holistic standpoint. Prayer and meditation can help to transform your thoughts to more positive, can do thoughts.

Like I stated above, we are not just the body, nor are we just the mind and spirit. We are a whole being: **Body, Mind and Spirit.** Therefore any desired changes need to address all three tiers if we want to be successful.

Mind

Since every change begins in the mind and in your thoughts:

- You've got to think about the change you desire. Think about it long and hard.

- Don't rush into your decisions because the choice you make, the decision you make, will be long-term. It will be for the long haul.

- It's okay NOT to embark on a new health journey in January when everyone else is on the bandwagon.

- Work on preparing your mind for the change.

- You may need to **pray** and seek guidance. You may need to **meditate** and seek guidance as you visualize the change you want.

- You may need to hire a **Lifestyle coach** or a **Health/Fitness coach** to help you to work through any ambivalence, doubts, and fears that you have.

MIND and MINDSET matter when it comes to weight loss.

My friends, you may ask me why you should lose those extra pounds and keep them off for good. Why shouldn't you just keep enjoying those delightful treats that you've grown to love over the years. Why not continue to binge on your favorite shows that you're so in love with? Why should you get up off that sofa and move?

My answer is that you've got to **find your "WHY"**.

Losing weight and keeping it off for good is not just about how you look..although that's very important. It's not just about how you feel, although that's very important.

Obesity is responsible for most of the Chronic health issues that plague Americans and people all over the world. Chronic debilitating health issues such as memory and mood disorders, diabetes and heart diseases. Obesity is responsible for some cancers such as colo-rectal cancer, which is one of the leading cancers in the US right now. Add to the list strokes, heart attacks, sleep apnea, and kidney diseases. Obesity can contribute to depression, anxiety, sleep disorders, and breathing problems, as well as gastric issues such as GERD, H pylori, constipation.

Menopausal issues, joint pains and stiffness, and the inability to conduct the activities of daily living are common. Many suffer from low self esteem due to being overweight. Folks feel helpless and frankly hopeless at times because they have tried all sorts of diets and fitness plans only to quit out of frustration because they are not getting the results promised or expected quickly enough.

Many books have been written detailing the many health risks connected to obesity and its deadly effects on our bodies and our mind.

So, it's important for you to first determine your "WHY". Why do you want to lose the excess weight and keep it off?

As I wrote in my first book, *Eat Sleep Meditate. A Nurse's Guide to Health in 2020*, I suffered with many of the health issues that I listed above.

I was diagnosed with a life-threatening heart disease called Cardiomyopathy. I was unable to breathe and had very low energy and palpitations daily. Drugs such as beta blockers, ace inhibitors and aspirin were of no use. My cardiologist told me that I might die if I was unable to get a heart transplant. The many side effects of the drugs made me feel sick, dizzy and weak everyday.

At the same time, I sank into deep depression and was full of anxiety. I was unable to sleep at night. Many nights I woke up after three hours, unable to go back to sleep. Like a clock, my body and mind would suddenly awake at 2 am, feeling wired, but tired and exhausted at the same time.

I was 38 years of age when this nightmare started. One year later, I had a heart procedure done to correct the irregular heartbeat/ arrhythmia, which my doctor stated was due to an electrical issue with my heart. That was successful. My electrophysiologist (a medical doctor who specializes in treating cardiac problems involving electrical activity and arrhythmia), instructed me to flush my many pills down the toilet, start walking at least 30 minutes daily, eat healthily, eliminate caffeinated drinks, get adequate sleep and decrease my stress levels.

Out of desperation to reclaim my health, and frankly, my fear of death at such a young age, I immediately started working on the doctors orders. At that time I had two young children and a husband to live for. I needed to be able to raise my children and ensure that they grew up and succeeded in life.

My many health issues spanned over 12 years or so. You see, although I had a wake-up call with my life-threatening heart disease, I still vacillated about the tough choices that were necessary to bring about total healing of my body and mind. I suppose one could say that I was ignorant or not convinced. Perhaps I could say that I was addicted to an unhealthy lifestyle, one that is not easy to unlearn.

During the 12 year span, I suffered with GERD, H Pylori, severe bloating and constipation. Pepsid, Zantac, Nexium, Prilosec worked for a brief while. I slept sitting up in an effort to decrease the acid reflux. My gastroenterologist was concerned, stating that chronic acid reflux is a risk factor for esophageal cancer, but he had nothing to offer but drugs. Multiple endoscopies confirmed H Pylori for which the treatment protocol was antibiotics and h2 blockers such as pepcid and the purple pill (nexium).

Needless to say, I was aware of the detrimental side effects of these drugs, but out of desperation I kept taking them. The constant nausea and abdominal cramps I experienced. The headaches and constipation and even the reflux were side effects of the nexium. The pepcid had its own set of negative side effects which I experienced. Trouble sleeping, joint and muscle pain, tiredness, dizziness and feeling faint.

Menopause came to me at about the age of 40. I experienced perhaps every menopausal symptoms known to women.

- Headaches
- Nasal congestion
- Trouble breathing
- Palpitations
- Night sweats
- Hot flashes
- Severe bloating and gas
- Nausea
- Irritability
- Weight gain
- Loss of sex drive
- Hair loss
- Dry skin

- Dry eyes

- Plantar fasciitis

- Joint and muscle pain

- Severe food and environmental allergies

So you asked me WHY did I choose to gradually transition to a Holistic healthy lifestyle?

The answer is that I was desperate for my life, my health. I was desperate to be around for my children and my husband. I was desperate to feel well, to look in the mirror and see a woman of hope looking back at me.

Over the years my "why" has changed and evolved. I am now 60 years of age and I find that it is just as imperative for me to do whatever is necessary to stay fit and healthy. This is because it can be a bit harder to lose the weight and to keep it off as we get older. My "why" is now to age healthy and fit, to look my best, to avoid blood pressure, cholesterol and diabetes drugs. To be fit enough to run around with my grandchildren, to look and feel attractive as I age. So our "whys" sometimes change or evolve.

My question to you is what is your WHY?

Why do you want to lose the excess weight?

Why do you want to get healthy?

Why do you want to feel good?

Why? Why? Why?

You've got to identify your WHY!

24

I have been asked during interviews if the transition to a Holistic Healthy Lifestyle and sustained weight loss was easy and quick. Absolutely not!

The transition to a healthy way was slow and steady with many setbacks, many mess-ups. Each time, I would reset, refocus and restart.

Mindset is the key to successful, sustained weight loss.

By the way, if you focus on weight loss alone, it is almost a guarantee that you will become frustrated and give up. Focus on a healthy lifestyle. Weight Loss is a byproduct of a healthy lifestyle. Eat healthy, home cooked meals. Exercise regularly, make sleep a top priority, reduce your stress level and enjoy life. This is the Holistic lifestyle that will lead to sustained, stress-free weight loss.

Now that you've identified your WHY, how do you begin?

- You may need to hire a personal trainer/fitness coach or a health coach.

- You may need to join a health club or a gym.

- You may need to hire a nutritionist.

These professionals can be quite helpful to help you to work out a system that is workable for you. They may be helpful to help keep you accountable.

- Consider linking up with other like-minded persons with similar health and fitness goals.

- Find co-workers or family members to exercise with and have healthy lunch swaps.

- There are multiple health and fitness experts, including physicians, physical and occupational therapists, nutritionists, health advocates like myself, who have your health, weight and wellness at heart, and provide videos, talks, seminars, webinars, exercise, diet and health tips.

- You can follow and subscribe to our websites, YouTube channels, Instagram, Facebook and other social media platforms where you will be notified when they drop a new video, is going live or when they send out a new health and wellness blog and newsletter.

- Consider joining a Facebook health and wellness and or weightloss group. Many of them are free and you can find tips in each that you may tweak and tailor to fit your specific goals and needs. I have a Facebook group called THE DOCTOR IN YOU. This group's goals are to help to encourage, motivate and inspire each member to incorporate the Healthy Holistic Lifestyle as part of their personal lifestyle. We share healthy recipes, eating tips. We share our exercise pictures and videos, as well as tips regarding sleep, stress management, fun and nature. Live videos are often done which gives the members an opportunity to participate and ask questions.

- Find a trusted friend and ask him/her to hold your hands. To hold you accountable. Someone who will listen but will love you enough to be tough. That person is me for some of my friends and my sisters. I am sometimes gentle with my approach; sometimes I am frank. Their feelings are initially hurt, but they usually thank me later for being open and frank with them about their health. Oftentimes the change we talked about comes years, months or weeks after the conversation. Be open to suggestions, guidance and corrections from those who love you and have your best interest at heart.

It is very important to develop a plan to stay consistent and motivated.

Discipline is the main ingredient to staying consistent and motivated.

Have a Plan:

- What days will you exercise?

- What type of exercise will you do and for how long?

- What will you eat for breakfast, for lunch, snacks and dinner?

- Do some research to see what healthy foods you can have that are not very high in calories. Some foods such as nuts and potatoes are healthy but high in calories. Do the homework, do some research to see how much of these foods you can eat without blowing your weightloss goals.
- A food journal might be beneficial as you track what you eat each day and make the necessary adjustments to fit your specific needs. This is where a nutritionist or a health and fitness coach may come in handy.

- Where can you find healthy, tasty recipes that you can prepare at home in a short amount of time? My book *SHEIR (Simple Healthy Easy Inexpensive Recipes* has over 100 recipes that you can whip up in your kitchen in less than 30 minutes). There are many cookbooks, cooking shows, and cooking videos that offer healthy recipes.

After the plan:

- Start to implement your plans.

- Start slow and build up.

- Stick with it!

- If and when you mess up, just hit that reset button and begin again

Mondays are my reset days. Mondays are when I get to Reset Refocus and Restart.

Typically on the weekends I eat a little more than I do during the week. I may even eat some foods such as ice cream or a piece of cake on the weekend, trying not to do this in excess, knowing that on Monday, I get to reset and restart. No guilt, just hit that reset button.

With time, you will find that the Healthy Lifestyle that you've been practicing and tweaking and figuring out has now become YOUR normal way of living. It is no longer stressful and you embrace and actually enjoy the new and improved you.

Don't sweat the small stuff

- Rome was not built in a day.

- You will not lose the excess weight overnight.

- Run from any weight loss program that promises quick weight loss. Quick off Quick on!

- It takes time and effort to unlearn the unhealthy way of eating.

- It takes time and effort to learn a new way to eat healthy.

- It takes time to figure out how to incorporate exercise in your busy schedule.

- It takes time to figure out what exercise you like, where you will exercise, when and how long you will exercise.

- It takes time to get used to getting up a little earlier to get your exercise in.

- It takes time and effort to plan and prep your healthy meals ahead of time.

- It takes time. Be gentle and patient with yourself.

Each time that I choose to eat something unhealthy, I remember my WHY and I get back on track.

Each time that I skip my exercise, I remember my WHY and I get back on track.

Each time that I stay up late doing whatever I do when I am up late (perhaps for you it is watching TV till late, or posting on social media or hanging out with friends) I remember my WHY, and I get back on track.

Each time that I am tempted to drink juice or coffee instead of water, I remember my WHY, and I get back on track.

Each time that I get back on track, Reset, Refocus and Restart, I am developing *Discipline* and *Consistency.*

When I feel like skipping my workout or eating unhealthy foods, I am reminded by someone that I follow on YouTube or Instagram or someone in my Facebook groups to get back on track and stay the course.

I am reminded that there are others that are watching me and holding me accountable.

These people keep me *Motivated.*

Once you develop *Discipline* through daily practicing,

Once you develop *Consistency* as you practice, reset, refocus and restart,

Once you identify and regularly connect with those who motivate you (like myself for example), the rest is history,

You then become the *Master of your health.*

You become and remain the healthiest version of yourself.

The stress no longer exists.

You become one with your new rhythm

This is what has worked and is still working for me.

The hard truth

As with any change, the hard truth is that ultimately YOU have to make the decision.

As with any change, motivation alone is not enough. You must practice discipline. You must be consistent. You must put the work in if you want to get the results!

As with any change, it all begins and ends with YOU.

There are no quick fixes or magical potions.

It begins and ends with you.

Losing weight and keeping it off for good require changes, and only YOU can make your changes.

Motivation is important, but what keeps you going?

What gets you to the finish line is *Discipline* and *Consistency* which comes with **Commitment and Practice.**

The mind is powerful throughout the weight loss journey.

We fix our weight by first healing our mindset.

Long before you make the firm decision to get on the weight loss lifestyle, start thinking about the journey.

- Get a blank book to journal.

- Set some short-term and long-term goals and write them down.

- Spend time with those goals. Think about them often.

- Feel the feelings of accomplishing that ideal weight and keeping it off permanently.

- Imagine yourself in those new clothes. How do you feel?

Your weight loss goal should be realistic yet somewhat challenging. For example, if your ideal weight loss goal is 60 pounds, this is not going to happen in 3 months. Be realistic. Perhaps the goals should be to lose 60 pounds in 2 years. Or to lose 1 pound per week.

It is unhealthy to lose weight rapidly and that way is usually unsustainable.

Small steps that are taken consistently become big steps.

Never compare yourself to others. Especially with social media, it is very easy to compare yourself to others. Everyone is on their own individual journey.

- Start where you are.

- Never compare yourself to others. We are all on our own individual journeys.

- Everybody was a beginner at one time. In the beginning, your goal is not so much about weight loss, but about building new habits that will be the foundation of your new healthy lifestyle.

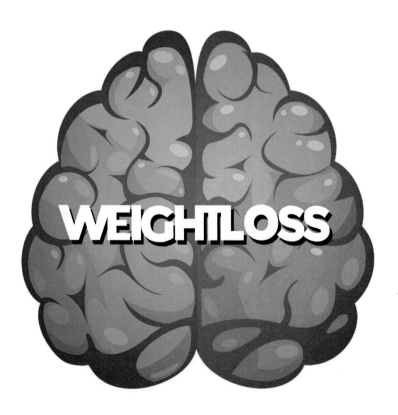

The Scale
Point to consider: For weight loss, the scale can be your best friend.

You are the one responsible for your health.

You are the one responsible for your journey.

Change begins and ends with YOU!

One way to be accountable to yourself is by weighing yourself regularly. **Daily weight** is actually a great idea.

The goal is not to beat up on yourself if and when you gain a pound or two, but to motivate you to make the necessary adjustments to your

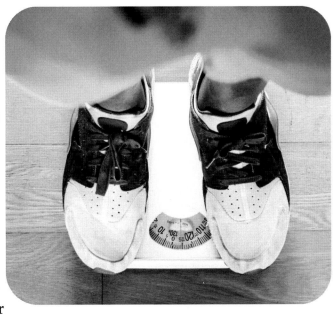

diet and perhaps your exercise, in order to drop that extra pound or two that you put on over the holidays or weekend.

Remember
- Mindset matters. Make a firm decision to do whatever it takes to lose the weight and keep it off for good. Start where you are.

Testimonial

"Good morning, I was thinking about you when I left the gym today. I think it is funny because a lot of people that don't work out say, "oh it's easy for you because you work out a lot to get up and go to the gym." I can honestly say that most days I am kind of dragging myself out of bed. Who wants to wake up at 5:20 in the morning to go work out? But the reality is that it's a commitment just like anything else. It's a lifestyle. If we could decide that we don't want to go to work just because we're tired, or we don't want to take care of our kids just because we're tired, we would never do what we have to do. It is a responsibility. Working out is also a responsibility to live a healthy lifestyle." (my son, Marlon Campbell)

Mindset matters!

You need a **Can Do Mindset.**

You need a **Committed Mindset.**

You need an **I will not give up Mindset.**

You need an **I will give it my best shot Mindset.**

You need an **I'm in this for the long haul Mindset.**

You need an **I will show up Mindset.**

You need an **I will fix my eyes on my goal and stay Focused Mindset.**

You've got to be desperate enough to make this work for you. You've got to be hungry enough for the end result of **sustained weight loss and reversal of health issues!**

Spirit

"Mindfulness is a type of meditation in which you focus on being intensely aware of what you're sensing and feeling in the moment, without interpretation or judgment. The Mayo Clinic defines mindfulness as "breathing methods, guided imagery, and other practices to relax the body and mind and help reduce stress."

Mindfulness and meditation help us to manage our stress levels. Excess stress often leads to overeating and we are inclined to grab that unhealthy snack when we are overly stressed. Some are also inclined to drink more alcoholic drinks when the stress becomes overwhelming. Alcoholic drinks can be quite high in calories which add up and can derail your weight loss goals.

Here are a few ways to incorporate mindfulness to help you to manage that stress so that you may succeed on your health journey and weight loss goals:

- Set aside 10 minutes each day to be still and quiet. Turn off the devices and just sit with your thoughts. Whatever thoughts come to you, be they good or bad, negative or positive, acknowledge them. Breathe.

- When you feel overwhelmed and anxious, close your eyes, take a few deep breaths, and relax.

- Try to focus on the task at hand. For example, if you are having your lunch, focus on every bite and enjoy it. If you are playing with your kids, be present and engage with them. When your mind wanders, return your thoughts to playing with your kids.

- Be kind to yourself. Treat yourself the way you treat others with kindness, patience, and love. Be gentle with you. Accept yourself. Try not to judge yourself.

- Go for a slow walk in the park or garden. Listen to the birds. Watch the squirrels. Be present with them.

Meditation

Managing stress is crucial to winning the war on weight loss.

It's quite normal to experience some stress on a daily basis, however, uncontrolled chronic stress can derail any weight loss goal. When we are chronically stressed out, the adrenal glands secrete excess cortisol which can promote overeating, which can lead to weight gain or difficulty losing the excess weight.

How do you manage stress?

- Meditation, Mindfulness and Prayer help.

- Plan ahead. Write a to-do list for everything. Check them off as accomplished.

- Prioritize. Some things can be rescheduled, postponed, or perhaps canceled.

- Solicit help from friends, family, or paid services.

- Journal how you feel.

- Speak to a therapist or nutritionist.

- You may need to **pray** and seek guidance. You may need to **meditate** and seek guidance as you visualize the change you want.

Body

Start slowly and build up. Oftentimes we go on radical quick weight loss programs. Drinking shakes, taking diet pills, eating next to nothing, and suddenly eliminating everything that we've grown to love over the years. This doesn't work.

Start to cut back slowly and gradually. Never totally cut out things suddenly. Even unhealthy foods. Cut back slowly. Go from 6 donuts to 5, then 4, and so on.

Whenever we completely and suddenly remove the foods we've learned to love and enjoy, our brain craves them.

When I was transitioning to a primarily plant-based diet, it took at least six months to do so, and I would often revert to heavy meat eating. I had to unlearn that old way and gradually learn the new way I wanted to eat. Everything takes time to unlearn and learn.

You could treat yourself to the goodies you like such as ice cream, donuts, or whatever your favorite treat is on the weekend, then reset on Mondays. I don't worry too much about eating super healthy on Saturdays, especially if I'm going out. Whatever I feel like eating, I eat (within moderation of course).

Come Monday, **I reset, refocus, and restart,** and I do it over and over and over again.

Meal Prep

Meal Prepping is a key element of successful, sustained weight loss. Plan ahead to succeed.

- Make a shopping list and stick to it. Only buy what you want to eat. If you buy a treat, only buy one. If you buy 6 donuts, you're going to eat all 6. If you buy one donut, there is only one donut to eat. Get the point?

- Shop in the periphery of the grocery store. This is generally where the healthier fresh, whole foods are. The middle aisle is generally packed with unhealthy, empty calories, canned, sugary foods that can derail your diet and keep the weight on you.

- Buy a lunch bag and a few to-go glass containers. Buy a few mason jars.

- Cook your meals for the entire week on your day off. Pack your lunch for the entire week in your to-go containers. Freeze them. Grab one each morning.

- Make enough vegetable salads in advance. Pack your salad in mason jars, enough for the week. Make sure the lids are sealed. Do NOT add your salad dressings until you are ready to eat your salad. Store in the back of your refrigerator. Perfect grab-and-go lunches, ready in less than 15 minutes.

Calories

Food for thought: Calories do matter. Not all calories are the same.

By eating a well-balanced diet, mostly plant-based, eliminating or minimizing processed foods, sugar, and artificial sweeteners. Minimizing meats, processed meats, and processed poultry. Drinking plenty of water. Watch the amount of protein, carbohydrates, and fats you consume, you're able to balance calories in and calories out.

In order for weight loss to happen, we must burn more calories than we eat or eat fewer calories than we burn.

Calories do matter!

Calories in=Calories out results in a stable weight

Some say calories do not matter and that calorie counting is nonsense, a waste of time. It has been my experience over the years that calories DO count when it comes to losing that weight and keeping it off.

Note: Remember that calories come from Fats, Proteins, and Carbohydrates, not just carbs as we are often led to believe.

- When the number of calories you consume equals the number of calories you burn, you will maintain a stable weight.

- Remember that in order for you to lose weight, there has to be a calorie deficit. That is, you must eat fewer calories than you burn, or you must burn more calories than you eat.

- Since calories come from Fats, Proteins, and Carbohydrates, weight loss will occur when our Fat calories, Protein calories, and carbohydrate calories intakes are less than the calories we burn through physical activities and other metabolic processes.

- Calories from donuts, pizza, white bread, flour products, cheese, sodas, fried foods, french fries, hamburgers, sweet drinks, cookies, crackers etc., are not the same as calories from wild rice, potatoes, quinoa, roots, carrots.

- Calories from processed foods will derail your health and weight loss goals.

- Calories from nutrient-dense foods such as wild rice, potatoes, legumes, nuts, grains, vegetables, and seeds are linked to a longer life and lower risk for chronic diseases such as cardiac diseases, hypertension, diabetes, obesity, arthritis, and even some cancers.

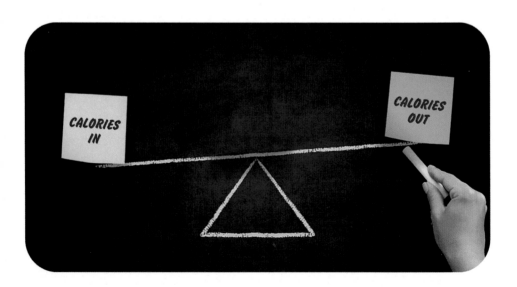

No Starving!

Eat enough food. Never starve yourself.

It's WHAT you eat

When you eat

HOW MUCH you eat

I never starve myself, except of course when I am fasting. (I will address fasting as a way to lose weight and keep it off for good later in this book.)

- You can eat to your satisfaction and still lose weight. It is all about what you eat.

- Not every calorie is the same.

- A cup of wild rice is not the same as 2 donuts.

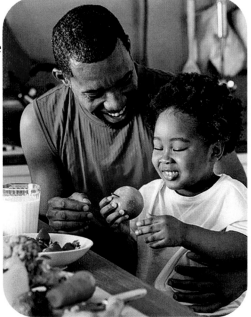

What you eat matters!

- **Aim to eat real whole foods:** Fruits, Vegetables, Nuts & seeds, Roots, Legumes, grains

- **Choose lean meats such as chicken, fish, and eggs.** (I eat a primarily plant-based diet, minimizing anything that is processed or not whole food plant-based.)

- **Learn to cook simple, wholesome, healthy meals.**

Processed Foods

Minimize processed foods. What are processed foods? A few examples of processed foods are:

- Breakfast cereals

- Cheese

- Canned foods

- Bread

- Pastries such as cakes, cookies, donuts, sausage rolls, pies

- Processed meats such as Ham, salami, turkey, sausage, bacon (yes even turkey bacon),

- Ready to eat microwaveable meals.

- Sodas, juices, milk drinks

Processed foods are less healthy because they usually have additives such as sugar and salt.

Eating processed foods can lead to you eating more salt and sugar than you should without being aware of it, thus derailing your health goals. (Read labels and avoid buying if the sugar and salt content are high.)

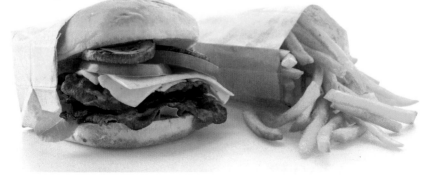

Breakfast

Start your day with a healthy, wholesome breakfast.

- Fruit smoothies generally have too much sugar and can lead to sugar cravings.

- Eat the whole fruits instead.

- Healthy meat proteins such as eggs, coupled with veggies such as peppers, onion, garlic, tomato, mushrooms, and green onion are often a hit with many folks. This is filling, low calories, nutritious and tasty. Make an omelet.

- My favorite breakfast is Oatmeal Bowls. Quick oatmeal has very little fiber, so I opt for old-fashioned or steel-cut oatmeal that can be cooked overnight, and the extras stored in the refrigerator for future use. Fiber-rich foods help to keep us feeling full longer. Top up your oatmeal with fruits. I love berries and apples, add chia, hemp, and flax seed powder. Sprinkle green powder such as spirulina, moringa, or dandelion greens powders. Or try a handful of walnuts or favorite unsalted nuts. Cinnamon, nutmeg, or cayenne pepper powder are also healthy choices (skip the sweetener). I find oatmeal bowls to be filling and will hold me for 4 to 6 hours. They are nutrient-rich and won't spike blood sugar.

- Plain unsweetened yogurt topped with fresh fruits and nuts can be quite satisfying, low calorie, and a healthy option for breakfast, lunch, and even dinner.

When you first start on your health journey, never skip breakfast! Perhaps eventually, if you choose to incorporate **Intermittent Fasting** into your lifestyle, you will probably skip breakfast. Eventually, you may find that you can actually skip breakfast because you do not feel hungry or have breakfast at lunchtime.

You will find a way that works for you if you keep trying.
Breakfast foods to avoid:

- Never eat fast foods for breakfast, this will derail your health journey for sure.

- Most packaged cereals are loaded with sugar and salt for taste and to preserve.

- White bread

- Bagels, croissants, muffins, and cupcakes

- Pancakes and waffles

- Breakfast pastries and breakfast bars

- Fruit juice

- Flavored yogurt and low-fat yogurt

- Processed meats such as bacon, sausage, and ham.

- Biscuits and gravy

- Pre-made smoothies, sugary coffee or sugary tea, hash brown patties.

These foods are packed with calories, fats, and refined carbohydrates and will most certainly cause your Health journey to be more challenging, often leading to frustrations and giving up.

Healthier Breakfast choices:

- Omelet with spinach, onions, tomato, peppers, eggs, and potatoes

- Multigrain toast with avocado and egg, sprinkle a little cayenne pepper

- Unsweetened, plain yogurt topped with fruits and nuts

- Vegetable smoothies with nuts and berries

- Oats, including overnight oats topped with berries, nuts, and green powder such as moringa, dandelion, or spirulina powders

- Apples with nuts or nut butter

Breakfast does not need to be traditional. Be creative. For example, I was out of oatmeal today. I have steel-cut oatmeal which takes at least 20 minutes to cook. I have cooked black beans and I also have walnuts. So I reheated the black beans, top with a handful of walnuts, sprinkle some cayenne pepper, and that was breakfast, with a few slices of watermelon. Healthy Leftovers can be a great breakfast choice.

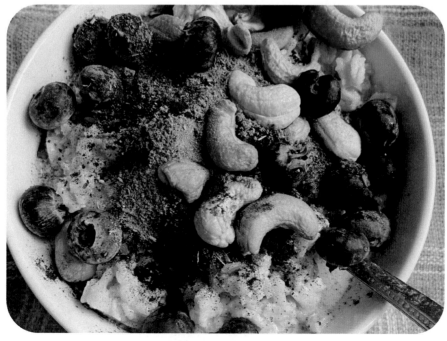

Oatmeal Bowl

Snacks

Snacks can be a game changer in one way or the other. Healthy snacks, such as nuts, fruits, carrots, and celery sticks are excellent. However, too many nuts can lead to excess caloric intake. As a general rule of thumb, about six nuts between meals, along with a few berries can calm that hunger or desire to eat. Wash that down with some water.

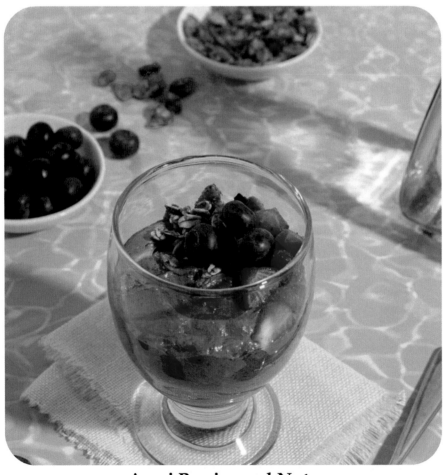

Acaci Berries and Nuts

Lunch

Lunch can be such a challenge for many as they dash to the cafeteria, conveniently located fast food restaurant, or favorite restaurant. These places usually offer healthy options, BUT who buys these? The smell of the french fries, hot dogs, hamburgers, fried chicken, chicken tenders, bacon, and fried eggs. The site of those big gulps becomes overwhelmingly tempting….and we succumb. We are only human…we have weaknesses.

Here is the cure for this: **Meal Prep!!**

- Make a shopping list.

- Cook meals for several days, perhaps the entire week on your days off.

- Pack your lunch in to-go glass containers with lids, enough for the week.

- Buy a lunch bag & a water bottle.

- In the morning before heading to work, grab one of your to-go lunches from your fridge, your water bottle, fruits, and a few nuts for a snack.

You have just set yourself up for **success** on your new Health Journey.

Stay away from **the cafeteria, fast food joints, or restaurants. Do not go with your friends and co-workers.** It is just too tempting, and you might not be able to withstand the temptation.

If you must eat at these places, try your best to make the healthiest meal choice that you can, but bringing your healthy lunch is a bulletproof way to succeed with lunch.

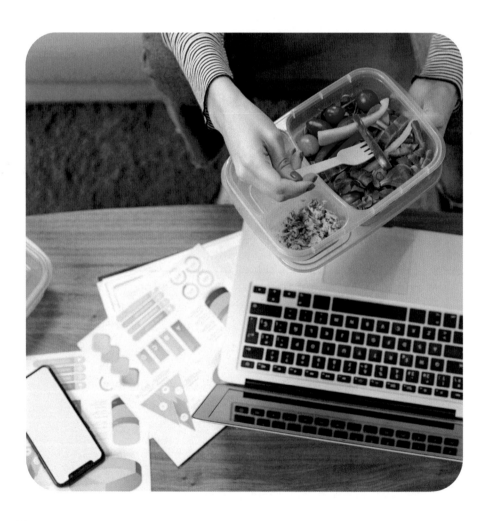

Dinner

Dinner can be a repetition of the Lunch idea.

If you get home from work later than 6 pm, it's probably a great idea to pack and bring your dinner to work with you and eat it at 6 pm. When you get home, try not to eat anything. If you must eat after 6 pm, go for some berries or ½ an apple since they are low in calories and are filling, along with a cup of herbal tea without sweetener.

Unless medical conditions prevent it, eat your last meal at least 3 to 4 hours before bedtime. Never go to bed with a full stomach. It's OK to go to bed a little hungry, in fact, it's a good practice, and you'll get used to it.

- Make dinner your lightest meal.

- Eat dinner early. If possible, eat dinner no later than 6 pm.

- Minimize the carbohydrates, fats and protein at dinner. Why? You will have little time to burn these calories before you go to bed.

- Go for salads minus the dressing and small portion of protein. The protein will help you to feel satisfied longer.

Intermittent fasting

Intermittent fasting (IF) is one of the most effective strategies for losing weight and keeping it off for good!

<u>A calorie deficit is a key to sustained weight loss.</u>

We need to either eat fewer calories than we burn OR, burn more calories than we eat.

So many assume that they can continue to eat whatever and whenever they want. They continue to eat high-calorie foods such as pizza, donuts, fried foods, sugary foods, excess meats, cheese and dairy, excess rice and potatoes, and so on, without consideration of the caloric intake.

Calories do matter, and calories come from proteins, fats, and carbohydrates…not just carbohydrates, as we are often led to believe. They don't realize that eating late in the evening or at night could be a huge factor that sabotages their weight loss goals.

Why is sustained weight loss so important?

That excess body weight that you carry around can have many negative effects on your health and wellbeing. If you are overweight or obese, you are at higher risk of developing health issues such as:

- Heart diseases

- High blood pressure

- Type 2 Diabetes

- Gallstones

- Breathing problems

- Some cancers

- Joint & Muscle pains

- Stroke

- Sleep problems

- Mental Health issues

- Low self-esteem

- Body image insecurity

- Fertility challenges

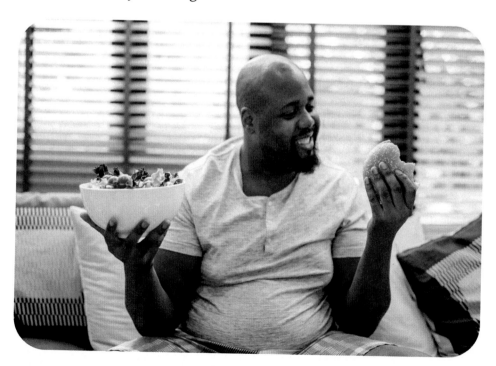

Research says that 95-97% of "Dieters" will regain all the weight they lost and then some within 1-5 years. Long-term weight loss is possible, BUT you must go about it the correct way. It takes work… don't be fooled by the illusion of quick & easy weight loss. Quick and easy is NOT sustainable.

Slow and steady is the best!

Adopting a sustainable Healthy eating pattern + regular exercise habits are vital for success.

Intermittent Fasting & Weight Loss

I have been using Intermittent fasting (IF) on and off for a few years as a tool to attain and maintain my ideal weight. This strategy has gained popularity in recent years, and many people are using it, along with regular exercise to achieve their sustained weight loss goals.

What is intermittent fasting? IF is an eating pattern that involves periods of minimal or no food intake. Although many use IF as a weight loss tool, there are health benefits to IF. Intermittent fasting can help to reduce, manage, or reverse health issues such as diabetes, Cardiac Diseases, and lowering of Cholesterol. It can help to improve blood pressure. Some research suggests that IF can help to decrease inflammation, improve sleep and even reduce the risk of certain cancers.

In recent months, I have fully embraced Intermittent fasting and regularly practice the 16:8 schedule, where I eat during an 8 hour window and fast for 16 hours. During my 8 hours of eating, I intentionally eat healthy, wholesome foods, avoiding processed, high-calorie foods, and drinking at least 64 ounces of fresh clean water.

Usually, I eat my healthy dinner no later than 6 pm. After 6 pm, I drink water or unsweetened herbal teas. I eat breakfast at 10 am or later. This gives me 16 hours of no caloric intake.

At first, it was a bit difficult to practice the 16:8 schedule, however, with time, this has become a norm for me, and I now feel very comfortable with it.

My stomach feels full and uncomfortable whenever I eat at night. With IF, I wake up the next day with my tummy feeling flat, I am not starving, and I actually exercise on an empty stomach without feeling low on energy, dizzy or faint.

I suggest that anyone who wants to consider IF do so slowly. Perhaps you can start by doing the 8:16 schedule, where you eat during the 16 hours and not eat for 8 hours at night. Gradually increase the fasting period and listen to your body. It is vital that you drink lots of water to stay well hydrated.

Intermittent fasting is not for everyone. Children, teens, pregnant women, people with diabetes or blood sugar problems, and those with eating disorders should definitely discuss any plans to start IF with their healthcare practitioner.

I have also found that IF boosts my memory and mental clarity.

Start slow and build up.

Physical Exercise and Sustained Weight loss

Even the least educated people are well aware that exercise and physical activity are important to attain and sustain a healthy state.

Physical exercise will not only help you to look good but as James Brown said, "Feel good" also.

Physical exercise offers many benefits including but not limited to:

- Improved brain health

- Weight loss and sustained weight loss

- Manage weight

- Reduce the risk of cardiovascular diseases, strengthening the heart

- Reduces the risk for Diabetes, some cancers and even dementia

- Strengthen bones

- Tones the muscles and improves flexibility

- Improves your ability to do your activities of daily living (ADL)

- Exercise helps to improve mood and boost energy

- Exercise is credited with improved sex life and sexual function

- Improve, manage and reverse high blood pressure

- Lower cholesterol

- Lower blood sugar

- Feel more energetic and strong

Exercise can be used to prevent, manage and reverse physical and even mental health issues such as depression, anxiety, anxiety, and inability to sleep. Exercise can improve cognitive function and boost self-esteem and self-confidence. Other benefits are relieving stress, and better quality, and quantity of sleep.

Exercise benefits our total Health and well-being.

Point to remember: All the exercise in the world will not lead to sustained weight loss unless we adjust our diet.

Here are a few tips to set yourself up for success:

1. Make regular exercise one of your top priorities.

2. Set specific **venue, days, and times** when you will exercise & stick to it.

3. Be reasonable with your expectations.

4. Make sure that your goals are not too high, or you could become discouraged.

5. Wear comfortable, weather-appropriate clothing and shoes that compliment your body.

6. Invest in a good pair of sneakers.

7. Start slowly and build up. The American Heart Association

recommends at least 150 minutes of cardio exercises per week. That adds up to 20 minutes daily or 30 minutes 5 days per week.

8. Break it up into bite sizes. 10 minutes in the morning. 10 minutes in the afternoon & 10 minutes in the evening is an option.

9. Select a convenient venue/place to exercise. If the gym or park is too far away or isn't open according to your schedule, then it's likely that you won't go.

10. What day and time will you exercise and for how long? For example, you might exercise every Tuesday, Thursday, and Saturday from 7 am to 7:30 am.

11. Never miss a workout, and if you do, make it up the next day. It will become a habit that you grow to love and enjoy. Never beat up on yourself if you do miss a workout session. Simply reset, refocus, and restart.

12. Invest in a Fitbit, or another tracking device to track your activity including steps.

13. Make use of any opportunity to increase your activity, such as taking the stairs instead of elevators. Parking your car farther away from the building. Walk to the neighbor or the store. Get up and move around while watching TV.

14. Subscribe to your favorite Youtube, Instagram, or any other social media Fitness channel. Follow them and get exercise ideas from them.

15. My biggest fitness investment this year is a set of bluetooth earpieces. This was a game changer for me. I tune in to my favorite YouTube exercise video, listening to the music as I jog and do my other workouts. Make it fun.

16. Add variety. Walk, jog, jump rope, skip. Do the ones you enjoy so that you don't get bored. Mix it up. This is where your favorite fitness guru comes in, you can get ideas from him or her.

17. Be sure to hydrate properly. If you are not well hydrated, you could feel low on energy and even dizzy.

18. Don't overdo things. If you are very tired, rest for a day and start again.

19. Find an exercise partner to workout with or just hold each other accountable.

20. Hire a personal trainer.

21. Join an exercise class.

Point to remember: Cardio alone is not enough!

Weight training and resistance training will help to maximize your workout.

Cardio is excellent for weight loss as you burn those calories during the workout. Resistance training and strength training helps you to build muscles, tone, and burn calories even when the workout session has ended. Combine both and you're well on your way to the smoking hot body you've been longing for.

Point to remember: As you make exercise your regular routine and habit, you will start to make healthier food choices. They just go hand in hand.

Never overdo exercise. You need a day or two for your muscles to recover after doing those weights and resistance training. For me, two days per week of weight training works perfectly. I choose Tuesdays and Thursdays for weight and resistance training. The other five days include cardio, such as jogging, brisk walking, and or jump ropes.

MAKE THE DECISION! BE INTENTIONAL!

- I will exercise every Monday, Wednesday, and Friday.

- You will exercise from 7 am to 7:30 am (walk, jog, jump rope).

- I will incorporate 10 minutes of upper body weight training on Mondays and 10 minutes of lower body weight and resistance training every Friday.

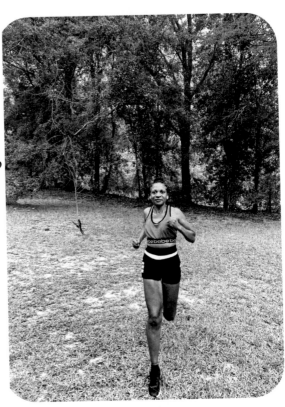

- I will exercise at the park near my children's school.

- I will set the alarm to get out of bed 30 minutes earlier, giving me time to get dressed and get to the park.

- I will understand that exercise without healthy eating is futile.

- I will understand that combining a Healthy diet + Exercise is best for sustained weight loss.

Personalize it! Make it yours!!

Start slow and build up.

You can do whatever you put your mind to.

Your mind dictates your habits & actions.

Cut out night eating! This is huge!!

Try this for two weeks and I guarantee that you will notice the difference in your tummy size and your waistline.

You will want to continue going to bed feeling a little hungry.

Eating late and eating at night leads to weight gain. Don't believe me? Try eliminating night eating for 2 weeks then reach out to me with the results.

Late eating leads to weight gain, but, if you Must eat at night for whatever reason, eat a bowl of salad, a bowl of steamed green veggies, and a small portion of protein and skip the carbohydrates and the fats.

- Drink more water. Thirst often presents as hunger.

- It's okay to go to bed a little hungry.

- Eat fewer calories than you burn.

- Burn more calories than you eat.

- Plan your meals ahead of time. Weekends are great for this.

- Set days and times for exercise in advance.

- Learn to cook healthy meals.

- Hire a personal trainer/Fitness Coach. Learn from them. Practice what they teach. Cut them loose if you cannot afford to keep them long-term. It might be a great idea to keep the Health and Fitness Personal trainer long-term if you are the type that needs someone to push you and keep you accountable.

- Hire a Health & Wellness Coach. They help to encourage you and keep you accountable.

- Restrict your caloric intake.

Reminder: The calories in food come from carbohydrates, proteins, and fats: A gram of carbohydrate has 4 calories. A gram of protein has 4 calories. A gram of fat has 9 calories.

Sleep

Get More **Sleep!**

The general recommendation is 7-9 hours of sleep per night. When you get adequate sleep, you'll feel more energetic and clear-minded and less likely to reach for that sugary food for that boost of energy.

When we sleep better, it is more likely that we will have more energy.

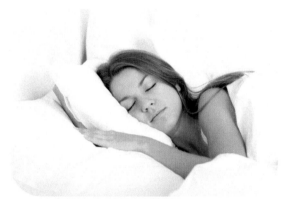

I cannot stress enough the importance of adequate sleep and decreasing your stress levels.

New research suggests that chronic stress can make you fat, not just because you stress eat, but that chronic stress may actually pump up the number of fat cells that we produce.

Chronic stress can lead to excess eating as a way to cope with the stressors. A way to make you feel better. Chronic stress can lead to increased cortisol levels which lead to the craving for unhealthy foods such as sugary foods, fatty and salty foods such as chips, pizza, donuts, and potato chips.

- Practice relaxation techniques such as Mindfulness, meditation, yoga, deep breathing, prayer, and journaling.

- Refuse to feed into the desire to eat unhealthy foods. Choose healthy all the time.

- Be consistent with your exercise. Exercise helps to decrease stress.

- Get 7-8 hours of sleep. Go to bed at the same time every night.

Insufficient and poor quality sleep is a major factor in weight gain, overweight, and obesity

- When we do not get adequate sleep, our bodies interpret that as stress. The excess stress leads to increased production of cortisol which leads to a craving for high fat and high carbohydrate foods

- Lack of sleep can also slow down your metabolism, which can lead to weight gain or inability to lose the excess weight

To sleep better at night:

- Dress comfortably.

- Dim the lights at least one hour before bedtime.

- Wear ear plugs to minimize noise.

- Turn off your devices at least one hour prior to bedtime.

- Hydrate early in the day. Yes, if you are not properly hydrated your sleep can be affected.

- Eliminate coffee and caffeinated drinks in the afternoon and evening.

- Try a noise machine.

- Take a warm shower or bath.

- Pray, Meditate, and Journal before going to bed.

- Same time to bed every night and the same time to wake up. Put a reminder on your phone.

- Turn off the TV and go to bed.

- Avoid heavy meals at least 3 hours prior to bedtime.

Let's summarize what we've learned:

- **Mindset matters.** Make a firm decision to do whatever it takes to lose the weight and keep it off for good. Start where you are.

- **Eat more veggies, fruits, and high-fiber foods.** 50% of your plate should be vegetables. Eat a raw salad with lunch and dinner. Remember that calories come from fats, protein, and carbohydrates. Avoid processed and unhealthy foods.

- Plan your meals ahead of time. Bring your lunch and dinner to work. Eat your dinner before leaving work.

- **Avoid night eating.**

- **Consider intermittent fasting.**

- **Weigh yourself at least once per week.** Daily weight works well for me. This will help to keep you accountable.

- **Get moving.** Do a minimum of 30 minutes of cardio exercise daily and include 2 days of strength training exercises. Stick with it. Discipline yourself. Stay the course.

- **Sleep for 7-8 hours at night.** Same time to bed, same time up.

- Reduce your stress level.

- **Hydrate with plenty of water.** Avoid sugary drinks and minimize coffee.

- **No starving yourself!** Eat enough of the right food. Never starve yourself.

- **Start slow and build up.** Never beat up on yourself. **Reset.**

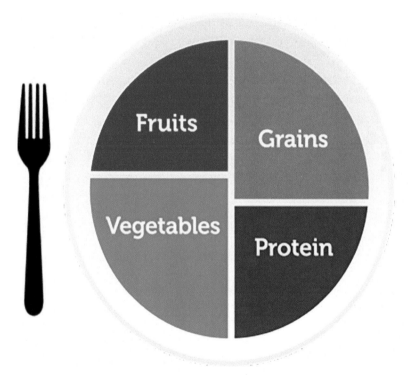

Eat Balanced Meals

Final Tips for Success

Here are 3 behaviors and habits that will help to set you up for success:

1. **Right Mindset:** Believe that it is possible for you to lose weight and keep it off for good. <u>Your mindset dictates your actions!</u>

2. **Right Discipline:** I will do whatever it takes to succeed. I will do the hard work. I will stick with it no matter what. When things get hard, and they will, I will not give up or give in! <u>Get out of your comfort zone.</u>

3. **Right Attitude:** Willingness to learn from others. Learn and challenge your current belief system about health, wellness, overweight, and obesity. <u>Be open to learning new fitness ideas.</u>

Here are 3 Questions to ask yourself:

1. What is health? Understand how your body works.

2. How can I make myself healthier?

3. What is the difference between good health and poor health?

Invest in your health!

Be willing to put in the work and stick with it. If it takes two years to figure things out and into a routine, then so be it. Quick weight loss is not sustainable. You are in this for the long haul.

Stay the course! Learn the rules to healthy living, leverage them, and use them to your maximum advantage!

RESET! REFOCUS! RESTART!
Every time!!

Mondays are great for **Reset, Refocus and Restart.**

Oftentimes, we overindulge on the weekends, picking up a couple of extra pounds as we nibble on this and that.

Don't be too hard on yourself. That is to be expected as we dine out with friends or family, as we let our hair down and have some fun.

Refocus, Reset and Restart

It's OK! Too much guilt can derail your goals. You might feel like a failure, giving in and giving up.

Simply **Refocus, Reset and Restart every time,** every Monday, every day as needed.

RESET.
REFOCUS.
RESTART.

Recipes
Eating our way to health

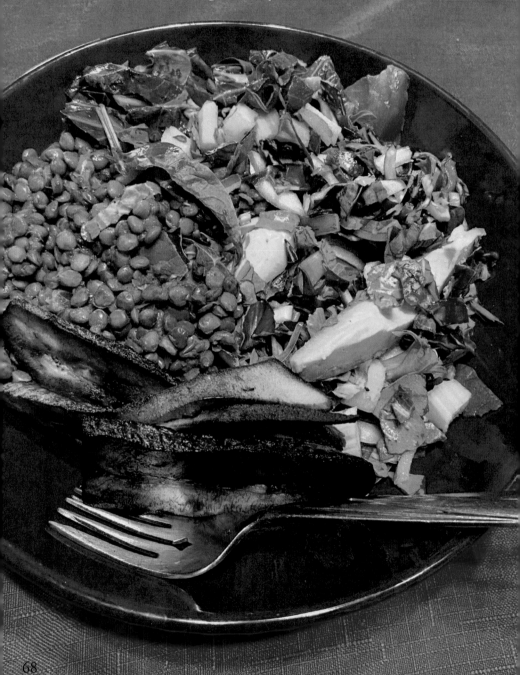

Breakfast

Ingredients
- 2 cups water
- 1 cup old fashioned oatmeal
- 1 tablespoon mixed seed (flax, chia and hemp) grind into powder
- Handful berries (blueberry, black berries, strawberries)
- 2 ounces unsweetened almond or soy milk
- Pinch ceylon cinnamon powder
- Pinch nutmeg
- ¼ teaspoon vanilla extract
- ¼ teaspoon moringa, dandelion or spirulina powder
- Handful walnuts or your favorite nuts

Cook oatmeal on medium heat for 5 minutes. Place in a bowl. Mix in almond or soy milk. Mix in flax, chia and hemp seeds powder. Top with berries, cinnamon, nutmeg, nuts and green powder, vanilla extract. Enjoy!

ONE POT MEAL: Mushroom, black beans, and potato curry

Ingredients:
- 2 tablespoons olive oil
- 1 onion chopped
- 1 large, sweet potato chopped into small chunks
- 4 ounces organic mushrooms washed and cut in halves
- 1 medium ripe tomato chopped
- 4 cloves fresh garlic chopped
- 1 cup cooked black beans (save the juice)
- 1 cup juice from the black beans
- 2 to 4 tablespoons hot Jamaican curry powder
- 1 pinch fennel seeds

Heat the oil in a large saucepan. Add the chopped garlic and fry till golden. Add onion and tomato, stir well. Add potato chunks, mushrooms, fennel seeds, black beans, juice from the black beans and curry powder. Stir well. Cover, bring to boil then simmer on low till the potato is tender, about 10 minutes. Serve with Rice.

Purple Cabbage Salad

Ingredients:
- 1 cup shredded purple cabbage
- ¼ thinly sliced sweet pepper
- 1 stalk green onion minced
- 1 small ripe tomato chopped tiny
- 1 Haas avocado sliced
- 1 cup chopped baby spinach
- Handful nuts

Mix everything together. Drizzle with raw apple cider vinegar with the mother and olive oil (or your favorite healthy salad dressing).

Watermelon Drink

Ingredients:
- 2 cups frozen watermelon without seeds and cubed
- ¼ teaspoons chopped ginger root
- ¼ teaspoon fresh mint leaves
- ¼ teaspoon lime juice

Blend everything together at high speed. Pour into glass and enjoy.

Uncle Donald's Natural Home Remedy for colds and flu

Ingredients:
- ¼ lime or lemon squeezed juice
- 1 teaspoon raw, organic, unfiltered honey

Mix the honey and lime/lemon juice till it becomes liquid. Drink twice daily.

My name is Marva Riley, a Registered Nurse, International Speaker, Holistic Health Advocate and author of the books Eat Sleep Meditate a Nurse's Guide to Health, SHEIR Recipe Book(-Simple Healthy Easy Inexpensive Recipes) and my new book Lose Weight & keep it off for good.

I advocate for a Holistic Healthy Lifestyle, which includes eating healthy, well balanced meals, moderate exercise, adequate sleep and mindfulness meditation , in order to equip our bodies to fight or prevent diseases.

A native of the Island of Jamaica in the West Indies, I immigrated to the US in 1989 with my two children and husband. In my late thirties, I was overweight and plagued with cardiomyopathy, a life threatening heart disease, severe depression and insomnia, H Pylori, GERD and paralyzing arthritic pain. I struggled with low energy and felt tired all the time. Low self esteem and a lack of confidence led to shyness and Social awkwardness. My doctor encourage me to lose weight in order to improve my health.

I tried the yo-yo diets, shakes, diet pills. I tried the gym. Oftentimes I would lose a significant amount of weight on these extreme diets, only to put all the weight back on as soon as I went back to eating "normal " food. With time and a bit of research, I found a Simple, sustainable system that helped me get to my ideal weight and stay there. I am 60 years of age and is enjoying my best health ever and has been at my ideal weight for several years.

Losing weight and keeping it off for good is Simple and doable. The key is to identify a system that works for you, practice it regularly, make it your own. This will take the stress out of it. You will then begin to enjoy the journey and it becomes an enjoyable lifestyle for you.

Will you allow me to show you how?

Marva

Made in the USA
Las Vegas, NV
16 March 2023

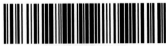

69204488R00045